CAREGIVING:

The Good, the Bad and the Blessings

Kelly Long Chappelle

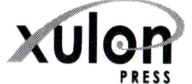

Copyright © 2016 by Kelly Long Chappelle

Caregiving: The Good, the Bad and the Blessings
by Kelly Long Chappelle

Printed in the United States of America

ISBN 9781498464093

All rights reserved solely by the author. The author guarantees all contents are original and do not infringe upon the legal rights of any other person or work. No part of this book may be reproduced in any form without the permission of the author. The views expressed in this book are not necessarily those of the publisher.

Scripture quotations taken from the New King James Version (NKJV). Copyright © 1979, 1980, 1982 by Thomas Nelson, Inc. Used by permission. All rights reserved.

www.xulonpress.com

Table of Contents

Dedication vii
Introduction ix
Chapter One – The Patients 11
Chapter Two – The Caregiver's Roles and
                Responsibilities 17
Chapter Three – Change 27
Chapter Four – Communication 37
Chapter Five – Care for the Caregiver 43
Chapter Six – Transition 51
Chapter Seven – The Blessings 65
Acknowledgements 71

Dedication

God truly blessed me with the most awesome parents a child could ever have, so I dedicate this book to them, Huey P. and the late Sandra Meades Long. I also dedicate this book to my son, Derrick M. Sewer, II, for his undeniable care, dedication, love and respect for each one of his grandparents.

Introduction

I share my story with you because unfortunately more of the earth's population is recovering, suffering or in treatment with life-altering illnesses, and therefore the need for caregiving has increased. The assistance and support a caregiver provides throughout various stages of the patient's life-altering illness will be instrumental to the patient. Prayerfully, my story will help caregivers understand what to expect, how to anticipate and deal with the challenges of being a caregiver as well as provide resources.

Additionally, my prayer for the caregiver is you are encouraged to walk the journey, find the energy to provide care and realize the strength God gives you to care.

CHAPTER ONE

The Patients

1 Timothy 5:8
"But if anyone does not provide for his own, and especially for those of his household, he has denied the faith and is worse than an unbeliever."

In late June 2007, my family and I sat in a cold, dark room at the hospital while the doctor explained my mom, who was brought to the emergency room by ambulance for back pain, actually had stage four breast cancer. The doctor told us that his examination revealed the cancer was metastatic and her kidneys had begun to fail and other organs had begun shutting down. Therefore, there was nothing they could do for her, but to try to make her comfortable.

This totally shocked our family because my mom had recently retired earlier that month from being an elementary school educator for twenty-nine years. So, instead of packing for the end of the school year, Mom also packed and moved boxes because of her retirement. She told us she felt back pain as a result of lifting and moving, and we had no reason not to believe her. However, the doctor explained the back pain Mom had endured was from her kidneys beginning to fail. Prior to receiving the news of my mom's life-altering illness, our family and her friends had never even seen her with a cold. Also, my mom exercised regularly and was a fairly healthy eater, so we never thought she would encounter cancer or any other life-altering illness.

Being an educator for so many years, my mom had many children other than her biological children, my brother and me. Somehow she managed to care for each of us like we were each her only child. Our house had a revolving door, especially on Sundays after church, mainly because Mom was known for her exceptional baking and cooking. We not only ate well on Thanksgiving, Christmas and Easter, but on every other occasion Mom could find to celebrate, such as birthdays, graduations, promotions, making the honor roll, a sporting victory, a birth, an engagement, healing, recovery and anything else she thought worthy to celebrate. No one minded all the celebrations because they were a chance to eat Mom's absolutely delicious food and scrumptious desserts.

Mom not only fed our appetites, she fed our souls by always finding a way to subtly share her spirituality and words of wisdom. Most important to Mom was her faith in the Lord Jesus Christ. She didn't have to preach about her faith because she lived it until she took her last breath.

The second most important to her was family. When my mom passed away, she was happily married to my dad for forty-nine years. Until God decided it was time for Mom to enter eternal rest on November 30, 2012, Mom lived what she called "a bonus round" after her terminal cancer diagnosis because she lived five years courageously physically fighting breast cancer as well as fighting passionately in support of causes for a breast cancer cure. For as long as I can remember, Mom supported organizations that fought for a cure for breast cancer. She volunteered, participated in walks, awareness campaigns and fundraisers with a great passion. Without knowing she would be personally affected by breast cancer, I guess Mom's participation in breast cancer awareness activities foreshadowed the battle she would endure in the future.

In November 2007, five months after my mom's diagnosis, my dad had a stroke. Prior to my dad's life-altering illness, he was a healthy, kind, strong, but quiet man with a wealth of knowledge and wisdom. Dad is an excellent provider, husband, father, grandfather, relative and friend. After retiring from the federal government, Dad couldn't sit still, so he went back to work in the graduate admissions office at one of the local universities. In addition to his second career, he spent his time exercising, traveling with Mom and serving at church and in the community. The most important thing to him, our family and friends is his constant presence and support to us all, no matter what his circumstances may be.

Since my dad also had a life-altering illness, I became my parents' caregiver. Every situation, whether good, bad or unpleasant, has something positive that can be gleaned. My family's life had drastically changed as a result of both of my parents' diseases; however, the good was I was in the position to become my parents' caregiver. My son was fifteen and able to provide support as well. I had a job where I was allowed to work my required hours in a flexible schedule, whereas my brother was unable to work a flexible schedule and he also had a new baby boy at home.

A year and a half after my dad suffered a stroke he had regained some independence. However, he was limited with what he was able to do, and therefore, I remained my parents' caregiver.

Chapter Two

The Caregiver's Roles and Responsibilities

Philippians 2:4

"Let each of you look out not only for his own interests, but also for the interests of others."

A caregiver has countless roles and responsibilities and those roles and responsibilities will not always remain the same. As the patient's needs change, you will have to adjust your caregiving roles and responsibilities in accordance to those needs. More than likely, the patient is not spending most of their time being treated in the hospital, but more of their time being treated at a doctor's office or at home, making the roles and responsibilities of the caregiver more important.

Usually the first responsibility of the caregiver begins after initial diagnosis of a life-altering illness because the patient will need guidance and support selecting providers for their care. The patient will face accepting the diagnosis and finding the strength to fight through the disease. As the caregiver, you will have to analyze, ask questions and assist with deciding on a team of providers who will provide the patient with quality care, respect and support. The following are some steps that you should take in selecting a good team of providers for the patient.

1. Talk to family members, friends, or co-workers to find out if they have any recommendations for providers. Also, call the local hospitals and medical schools for recommendations. If the patient is or was in the hospital when they received the diagnosis of their disease, ask the hospital staff for recommendations for medical care.
2. Don't stop with the first recommendation you obtain; call around to several different providers and consider your choices before making a

selection. Also, read the websites that rate doctors based on reviews from actual patients.

3. If their primary care physician diagnosed the patient, and they refer the patient to a specialist, still check them out. Unfortunately, some doctors may refer the patient to one of their friends who may not be the best doctor for the patient or a doctor that is not within the patient's insurance network. Please keep in mind the patient's primary care physician is usually the physician responsible for coordinating all of the patient's care, which should ensure they receive the best medical treatment for their disease.

4. Research to make sure the providers have the appropriate credentials and are properly licensed. You can do a background check by calling your state's medical licensing board and ask for a background check on the provider.

5. Also, check the hospital's or medical facility's cleanliness, quality and reputation.

6. If you have to find a surgeon, research how many times the surgeon has performed the procedure and their success rate.

7. It is important to discuss insurance plans with the providers. Besides ensuring the provider is covered under the patient's insurance, specifically you have to determine if the insurance covers all visits, medications, procedures, tests and treatments that are anticipated to be provided. Then contact the patient's insurance company to discuss coinsurance, copays, deductibles, referral procedures and other terms and conditions that may affect insurance coverage and the patient's care.

8. Good bedside manner is extremely important to the patient's care and well being. You don't want the patient to have a provider who will walk in the treatment room and not say hello and only begin to talk about themselves, deliver the diagnosis and then walk away without discussing the diagnosis. The patient needs to have a provider who is tolerant and will thoroughly explain the diagnosis and options for treatment. It is also important for you and the patient to have forbearance and wait an extra twenty or thirty minutes if necessary, to see the provider because the delay will most likely be due to the other patients who are being properly

The Caregiver's Roles and Responsibilities

cared for who were scheduled with an earlier appointment time.
9. To ensure the patient will be able to get proper care in case of an emergency, research after-care hours, after-hours contact information and emergency treatment procedures of the providers.
10. Research to see if the provider's approach to healing and treatment is consistent with the patient's beliefs, spirituality and other views.

Now that you have selected a good team of providers for the patient, it is important to remember that demonstrated support of the patient to the providers will help ensure better care because the providers will know they may be challenged if things are not progressing as the patient, patient's family or caregiver anticipated.

When the patient has to stay overnight in the hospital, that is not a vacation for the caregiver; it is another time where demonstrated support to the patient is required. It is important to understand the hospital and their actors. Fortunately, one of our family members is a nurse and assisted tremendously whenever I was confused, needed guidance or someone to speak the same language as actors in the hospital listed below.

1. A *hospitalist* is a dedicated in-patient physician who works exclusively in a hospital.
2. A *charge nurse* is in charge of a ward in a hospital.
3. A *RN* is a *registered nurse* who has graduated from a nursing program and has passed a national licensing exam to obtain a nursing license. A RN in the hospital administers medications, cares for wounds, conducts physicals and assists with coordinating the patient's care with providers.
4. A *LPN* is a *licensed practical nurse*. An LPN functions under the direction of an RN providing direct patient care.
5. A *patient care technician* will become the patient's best friend. A patient care technician will check blood pressure, heart rate, pulse and temperature. A patient care technician will assist when the doctor or nurse performs an exam. They also change bedding, help the patient bathe, shave or change clothes. When

walking is needed, a technician will help the patient walk to their destination. A patient care technician will ensure the patient receives meals on time and monitor food intake. If a patient is confined to the hospital bed, the technician will ensure bedsores or other skin problems are not an issue.

As a caregiver, you will have to learn how to do things that used to be done by health care professionals including home health aides such as administering medicines (including shots), bathing, dressing, feeding, grooming, oral hygiene, toileting, lifting and moving the patient, monitoring side effects and reporting concerns, issues or problems to the providers.

As a caregiver, you will be an administrative assistant, scheduling appointments, tracking prescriptions, ordering medical supplies, taking notes at appointments, handling health insurance issues and financial matters. Get to know the patient's pharmacist. You will need to ask if they will carry the patient's anticipated medication. Also ask if there are options if the patient's prescriptions are needed after the pharmacy is closed. There may be alternative treatments, herbs or supplements the patient has heard of and may want to try. However, the patient or caregiver should consult with the provider and pharmacist before the patient tries any of the alternatives.

As a caregiver, you will be a personal assistant, conducting tasks such as doing laundry, grocery shopping, household chores and maybe even some minor home repairs to name a few.

As a caregiver, you will also become a taxi service providing transportation to and from appointments. One of the characteristics a caregiver must maintain is punctuality. If your patient is late for an appointment, they may not be able to be seen by the provider or receive treatment scheduled for the day. Not only will the patient miss the appointment, but they may also incur a cost because some providers charge if you miss an appointment without cancelling at least twenty-four hours or more in advance. Most likely, the patient you are caring for does not move as fast as they did before being diagnosed with a life-altering illness. So, when scheduling appointments account for time to bathe, dress, groom, eat, take medicine, getting the patient from their home to the car and driving to the appointment. Even if you will not be driving the

The Caregiver's Roles and Responsibilities

patient, you will be coordinating their transportation because they will be transported by a family member, friend or non-emergency medical transportation service, so you must plan accordingly when scheduling the patient's pick up time.[1] Since there will be a lot of time spent traveling in a vehicle to and from appointments, make sure the patient has their favorite CDs, or download their favorite music to an iPod, iPad or cell phone so they can listen to music. Going to a doctor appointment, receiving treatment, taking a medical test or receiving a procedure, no matter how minor the procedure, may be stressful for the patient. So listening to their favorite music will not only pass the time but also relax them in their travels to and from medical appointments. If music will not be relaxing for the patient, provide them with puzzle books like Sudoku, crossword puzzles or word search. These puzzle books can be found at a dollar store or in the dollar section of Target. If puzzle books still don't provide relaxation,

---

[1] If you are insured by Medicare, they may cover limited, medically necessary non-emergency medical transportation to obtain treatment or to diagnose a medical condition and the use of other transportation method could endanger the patient's health. For more information, call 1-800-MEDICARE or 1-800-633-4227.

try a magazine about their favorite activity or sport or a book. Novels are sometimes hard for the patient to read because with so much going on in their lives, it is hard for the patient to focus on completing a novel. If music, puzzle books, a magazine or novel still won't provide relaxation, try giving the patient a journal and a set of pens to write.

As a caregiver, you will make mistakes, but do not dwell on those mistakes or feel guilty about them. Learn from the mistakes and move on because you have a lot of caregiving to do.

Chapter Three

Change

2 Corinthians 4:16-18

Therefore we do not lose heart. Even though our outward man is perishing, yet the inward man is being renewed day by day. For our light affliction, which is but for a moment, is working for us a far more exceeding and eternal weight of glory, while we do not look at the things which are seen, but at the things which are not seen. For the things which are seen are temporary, but the things which are not seen are eternal.

After the diagnosis of a life-altering illness, the patient's life will significantly change.

The patient may normally be a pleasant and positive person, but their diagnosis may leave them angry, frustrated, anxious, sad, guilty, depressed and/or scared about the changes they are about to go through. One thing you can do as the caregiver is research to find information about the disease the patient has been diagnosed with to ease the fear of uncertainty about the changes to come. If the person is normally cantankerous, brace yourself because usually as the closest person to the patient, the caregiver is the one who suffers the consequences of the patient's anger and frustration, simply because you are there. As a caregiver, you must learn to not take things personally. Mom was not happy about the changes to her life as a result of battling breast cancer, but she was a good patient who never complained, but thanked God each day for another day and focused on helping others the best she could as she had always done.

Dad too was not happy about the changes to his life as a result of suffering from a stroke; however, he was at times a challenging patient. Dad had an all-or-nothing mentality. He felt if he wasn't the man he used to be prior to suffering from a stroke, he couldn't provide or support his family and friends as he had always done. For Dad, I needed reinforcement from a few of his beloved family members who grew up with him and knew him well enough to know what to say to him to help me convince him that not being able to do some things he used to was better than not being able to anything at all. In addition, we had to convince Dad that his diagnosis did not prevent him from doing things to assist his family and friends; it only changed the way he was able to assist.

The patient's diagnosis may limit their ability to go places and do things they enjoyed or had to do, like cooking, driving, eating, working or participating in their favorite activities or sports.

Mom loved to bake and cook for her family and friends. So when her hands weren't steady enough, or her legs could not hold her up long enough to create her delicious meals and scrumptious desserts, she was frustrated. To compensate for Mom's absence in the kitchen, we would order carry out from her favorite restaurants or meals at home through delivery services, but soon this became frustrating for her as well because she missed eating a good home-cooked meal. In addition, when dietary restrictions became part of my parents' treatment plan, we needed to ensure certain ingredients in the food didn't have an adverse effect on their health. Mom's frustration was unsettling for me, so I decided I would get in the kitchen and cook, not bake, because there was no way I could try to master both. Even though Mom was not in the kitchen, she always made sure she was close to guide me along. She was such a good cook that she could smell when I had too much of one spice or seasoning and not enough of another when I tried to cook one of her specialties. This was exasperating for me, because it always took several iterations for me to get whatever I made to satisfy her taste. One of the side effects of one of the types of chemotherapy Mom received during her battle was the loss of taste, which was selfishly good for me because I only had to cook things one time instead of multiple times since during that time, she ate not for taste, but nourishment.

One of the places Mom loved to go was church. Church allowed her to do most of the things that were important to her: worship her Lord and Savior Jesus Christ, sing (she was a member of the choir), play the piano or organ (she was the keyboardist), teach (she taught Sunday school), bake and cook for church events and members, learn from Bible study and sermons, fellowship with other church members and coordinate church activities and events. So when Mom was unable to attend her church home of over thirty years, she was devastated. Prior to not being able to go to church because of her diagnosis, Mom had strong thoughts about attending bedside Baptist by watching church online or on television because she felt that you were detached from other members of the body and therefore could not gain all that church has to offer. Mom always said there was nothing like being in God's house and spending time with God's family. She often referred to Hebrews 10:24-25 when it came to going to church: *"And let us consider one another in order to stir up love and good works, not forsaking the assembling of ourselves together, as is the manner of some, but exhorting one another, and so much the more as you see the Day approaching."* The church I am a member of not only streams Sunday worship services live, but also their Tuesday night Bible study, which curtailed Mom's devastation about not being able to attend her church home. Especially since the pastor always acknowledged those watching online during the livestream by coming on before his sermon and thanking those watching online. The pastor also provides the scripture and sermon title at that time. An added bonus for Mom was the pastor included those streaming in his prayer prior to preaching his sermon. Another thing that eased her devastation was her deacon faithfully came to provide her with Communion when she was unable to attend their church home on first Sundays.

Traveling was a major part of my parents' life. I believe together they visited almost every state in the United States except Alaska and Hawaii. Further, I don't think there was a jazz festival that they missed between Montreal, Canada and Florida. Their life-altering illnesses significantly changed their travel itinerary. They still traveled, but only for special occasions and I had to accompany them. If we drove, a four-hour trip became a six-hour trip.

If the person you are caring for is susceptible to blood clots, they cannot be seated for extended periods of time, so you have to stop to allow them to stretch their legs. One of the side effects of medicines the patient takes may be a frequent trip to the bathroom, which also requires many stops on a road trip.

The patient's diagnosis may change their financial situation and/or employment. When diagnosed with a life-altering illness, there will be a change in the patient's financial situation, whether they are rich or poor. The patient will be responsible for co-payments, deductibles, prescriptions and medical supplies. They also may have to pay for transportation costs to and from medical appointments if a family member, friend or Medicare does not cover this expense. Since patients spend more time at home, their utility bills may increase, especially if the patient is using medical equipment that requires electricity.

If the patient is employed, a life-altering illness will definitely change their employment situation. The patient will probably want to work if they are able to do so to maintain their income and health insurance. Hopefully if able to work, the patient's employer will work with the patient to find ways for continued employment. For example, maybe telework or an alternate work schedule will be options. Or maybe the patient can develop a plan along with their employer that incorporates accommodations that will allow the patient to continue to perform their job. If the patient is unable to work, they should discuss with their benefits department about ways to continue health benefits such as short-term disability, long-term disability, long-term care insurance, Consolidated Omnibus

Budget Reconciliation Act (COBRA) or other options that their employer may have so that the patient may maintain health insurance.

Depending on the type of disease the patient is diagnosed with, their body may change both inside and out. Some of the observable changes may be that they walk slower, talk differently, their skin may change colors or be dry, weight gain or loss, rapid hair growth or loss, extreme fatigue, memory loss, crying, yelling, no patience, dizziness, sores that won't heal or loss of nails. Their physical needs may change as well. For example, if the patient used to be able to shave with a razor, they may need to use an electric razor now. If the person was a slow eater before, then most likely they will become a slower eater. Also, be sensitive to the foods and drinks you give the patient. If they are moving slower now, tea might not be a good idea. Things with acid like pineapple aren't a good idea either. Things that will settle in their stomach well and not keep them or you, the caregiver, running to the bathroom with them since they can't run at the moment are best. Try not to focus on the physical changes that the patient will endure. Focus on keeping the patient's spirits uplifted. Proverbs 17:22: *"A merry heart does good, like medicine, but a broken spirit dries the bones."*

The diagnosis may also change their personal relationships. Some of the patient's friends, coworkers and even family members may have a hard time visiting or talking to the patient now that they have a life-altering illness. Some people will be uncomfortable because they will not know how to talk to or act around the patient. Talk to the patient to find out what type of behavior and conversation they will appreciate so you as the caregiver can let people know what may be offensive or disturbing to the patient. When someone has a serious illness and his or her appearance is different as a result, it is unpleasant and can be depressing. However, keep in mind the patient has not changed from the person you have always known. The most appropriate way to deal with the patient is in the same manner you always have.

Chapter Four

Communication

Colossians 4:6

"Let your speech always be with grace, seasoned with salt, that you may know how you ought to answer each one."

Communication is different after a life-altering illness. As the caregiver you should keep the following in mind in regards to communicating with the patient.

Your patient has a lot of concerns, fears and thoughts running through their mind so accept they may need silence. A lot of conversation may annoy the patient and interrupt their thoughts, whereas silence may comfort them and give them an opportunity to talk about their concerns, fears and thoughts.

Focus on the patient. Pay attention to what your patient says as well as how they say it to determine if the patient needs you to listen or have a conversation. Whatever you determine to be the patient's desire, it is important to accommodate their need.

My dad always told me to look a person directly in the eyes when talking to them. His advice comes in handy for a caregiver. It is important to look the patient in the eyes when communicating with them to ensure the patient you are listening to them and they have your undivided attention and support.

It is not a good idea to ask your patient, "How are you?" Ask the patient a question about himself or herself that will provoke more than a one word answer and yield to a conversation where the patient can share how they are doing or feeling. However, position yourself mentally and physically to hear how the patient is doing and feeling because they may want to discuss death, pain or other uncomfortable things.

Even though you may have the patient's best intentions at heart, unless you are a professional, it is not a good idea to give the patient advice. The patient will more than likely benefit from you lending your ear rather than lending your advice.

Once family members, friends, coworkers, and neighbors hear about the patient's illness, the patient is more than likely going to be overwhelmed with phone calls, texts, emails and visits. As the caregiver, learn when the patient is too overwhelmed to respond and take over communicating until the patient can handle all the greetings and correspondence again.

For a lack of words, people may say to the patient, "you look good," even if the person has lost all their hair, had a significant amount of weight gain or loss or a change in skin color. Instead of saying, "you look good," say, "I enjoyed the time we were able to spend together today and hope to have the opportunity to spend more time with you again soon."

Unless you also have the same disease as the patient, do not say to your patient, "I know how you feel," or, "It will get better tomorrow." You won't know how they feel and you are not God and therefore cannot predict what will happen tomorrow.

James 4:13-15

Come now, you who say, "Today or tomorrow we will go to such and such a city, spend a year there, buy and sell, and make a profit"; whereas you do not know what will happen tomorrow. For what is your life? It is even a vapor that appears for a little time and then vanishes away. Instead you ought to say, "If the Lord wills, we shall live and do this or that."

While you are caring for the patient, if you feel like you are about to cry, leave your patient until you can get it together. If you have already started crying, tell the patient it is difficult to see them have to deal with this disease and leave your patient until you can get it together. The last thing you want to do is have your patient comforting *you* about *their* diagnosis.

Laugh and have conversations about things other than the patient's disease so everything in the patient's life is not consumed by their sickness.

Try to do as many things together as possible. If you used to play Scrabble or Checkers, play. If you used to go to the movies, go. If your patient is unable to go to the movies then there is cable, Netflix and

Redbox. If you used to shop, shop online if the patient can't physically go to the store. If you used to paint, scrapbook or do other arts and crafts together, continue to do them. The most important thing to remember is know how much activity your patient is able to handle. Accommodate the patient if they get tired and need to take a break while doing an activity. Also, if they need their private time, provide it to them.

CHAPTER FIVE

Care for the Caregiver

Hebrews 4:16

"Let us therefore come boldly to the throne of grace, that we may obtain mercy and find grace to help in time of need."

Just as your patient has needs, so do you, the caregiver. As the caregiver, not only do you have to care for the patient, you may have to go to work, take care of your family and maintain other responsibilities in your life. So it is important for the caregiver to take time to care for their needs and rejuvenate themselves to be able to emotionally and physically be able to take care of the patient. If you can't take care of yourself, you will not be able to take care of the patient. You will need to listen to your mind and body when they are telling you that you need rest. Do not feel guilty about needing rest and taking a break; caregivers need help too. Allow others to help you care for the patient. Many may want to help, but will not know how, so to help keep a list of things that will be helpful to you and allow yourself to have some relief from your caregiving duties. The list may include things such as: babysitting the patient's children, laundry, cleaning, cooking, minor household repairs, transportation or grocery shopping. If you have someone do things, first make sure they are capable of doing them. If your patient needs to be lifted or moved, you cannot have someone with their own physical challenges care for the patient in your absence, but maybe that person could do something else like read to the patient. However, make sure if the patient likes to read romance novels, they don't read a science fiction novel to them.

If someone grocery shops, insist on giving them a list. I had someone volunteer to grocery shop but the person lost the grocery list in their travels so they created their own grocery list. What they bought was appreciated, but unable to be eaten by Mom or Dad.

My mom loved green beans, so one of my friends took the time to cook green beans and homemade chicken noodle soup for my parents. Mom was elated and appreciated my friend's effort to bring over two of her favorite foods; however, this was a time when Mom could taste and was not only eating for nourishment, so the green beans were not to her liking, but the green beans did not go to waste because my son and I ate them. She and my dad loved the chicken noodle soup.

Mom had a wheelchair that had a loose wheel, which made it hard to push her in it, so a family member volunteered to fix the wheelchair. The day after the wheelchair was "fixed," Mom's niece took her to a doctor appointment and while she pushed Mom in the rain, the wheel of the wheelchair fell off which left Mom and her niece in the mud. Fortunately, my brother had stopped by on his way to work and was able to do a temporary fix. While my brother fixed the wheelchair, the ladies had to clean themselves off, therefore were not going to be on time for Mom's appointment for treatment. Fortunately, the oncology office was flexible and even though Mom was late, she was able to receive treatment that day. So make sure the repairs that need to be done on your list are done by someone who is not only willing to help, but capable. For those that want to help and cannot physically come to see the patient and provide you with relief, ask them to send letters and cards or send emails that can be printed to make the patient feel encouraged and supported. They may also want to mail books, CDs, DVDs, magazines, crossword puzzles, word find or Sudoku for the patient to use while in providers' waiting rooms or while receiving treatment.

Encourage the patient's family and friends to invite the patient out to enjoy things they have always done. The patient's time away will provide them with normalcy and you with some relief from your caregiving duties. Tell the patient's family and friends not to be discouraged if the patient declines an invitation and to please ask again. It may be that particular day that the patient is not up to the activity or outing.

The caregiver needs to have someone to talk to who is not close to the situation. This person should be someone who can provide an outlet for you from your caregiving duties. It should be someone who can take your mind off of the current situation and make you laugh.

Depending on how long you are a caregiver, you may have lost your passion for things you like to do because your life has been consumed with the patient's life-altering illness. However, you must find that passion again. If you like to do arts and crafts, make time to do so. If you like to go shopping rather than shop online, make time to do so. If you like to go to the movies, make time to do so. If you have a favorite television show you have missed because of your caregiving duties, record it and make time to watch the show. If you like to go fishing, make time to do so. If you like to take long scenic drives, make time to do so. If you like to exercise, make time to do so, although as a caregiver you are probably getting quite a bit of exercise. If you enjoyed getting pampering and lingering conversations at the barbershop or beauty salon, make time to continue to do so even if it is not at the frequency you are used to. Whatever activity you enjoyed prior to your patient's diagnosis, you need to resume that activity even if it is on a minimal basis. If not, find something else you can find time to do in its place because a break from caregiving is necessary.

Prior to becoming a caregiver for my parents, I took an annual extended weekend vacation—"a girl's trip." My parents encouraged me to continue to do so which was a blessing because when I returned, I was always refreshed, rested and rejuvenated to continue with work, caring for my son, my parents and other responsibilities. If you are unable to take a vacation, then try to find time for a staycation at a local hotel at least for one night. Or maybe you could stay at a friend's house for a night. Or if you have nowhere to stay, then spend the day away from caregiving and treat yourself and enjoy one of your favorite activities.

I love to swim, but rarely found the time to do so because after the time it would take to drive to and from the pool, shower and do my hair, too much time was consumed. Mom was always on fire for the Lord and as she battled breast cancer, her faith remarkably increased. Her faith got her through days, nights and hours of pain and suffering. Yet she never complained. Since I could not find time to swim, to take care of myself, I dove into the Word of God, as Mom always did because it helped her mind and soul so I thought it would help me as well. In between work, taking care of my family and performing my caregiving duties, I would find a place to park my car or when it got dark early, I found a Starbucks or Panera Bread and read the Bible before I began my caregiving duties.

I will share with you a few scriptures that I relied on heavily. You will need strength to handle the mental and physical challenges of caregiving. You also will need strength to manage your family, job and other responsibilities while being a caregiver. So when I needed strength, I read Isaiah 41:10: *"Fear not, for I am with you; be not dismayed, for I am your God. I will strengthen you, Yes, I will help you, I will uphold you with My righteous right hand."*

You will need comfort when things happen out of your control with family, your job and the patient. Prayerfully all these areas are not out of control at the same time but they may be and you will not have the luxury of crawling into bed and snuggling under a blanket to find comfort. So when I needed comfort, I read Psalm 34:18: *"The Lord is near to those who have a broken heart, and saves such as have a contrite spirit."*

You will get scared at times about what lies ahead for the patient you are caring for, so reading Psalm 23:4 should help you through times of fear and uncertainty: *"Yea, though I walk through the valley of the shadow of death, I will fear no evil; for You are with me; Your rod and Your staff, they comfort me."*

You will need to peace to deal with the patient's life-altering illness and the changes to the patient's life as well as yours. So when I needed peace, I read John 14:27: *"Peace I leave with you, My peace I give to you; not as the world gives do I give to you. Let not your heart be troubled, neither let it be afraid."*

If you have the unfortunate experience of watching the disease take its toll on the patient's body, mind and soul, you will need hope. When I needed hope, I read Revelation 21:4: *"And God will wipe away every tear from their eyes; there shall be no more death, nor sorrow, nor crying. There shall be no more pain, for the former things have passed away."*

CHAPTER SIX

Transition

---

2 Corinthians 5:1

"For we know that if our earthly house, this tent, is destroyed, we have a building from God, a house not made with hands, eternal in the heavens."

Doctors are not God; they are not able to determine how long the patient will live. When the patient's prognosis does not look good, it does not mean you or the patient should give up because transition does not always mean death. There are always new findings from research and new or different treatment plans that provide hope in controlling, if not curing, the patient's disease. Regardless of the prognosis, it is important as the caregiver to help the patient have the best quality of life possible.

In August 2012, Mom's oncologist advised my dad, brother and I there was not much more they could do for Mom. Her cancer had metastasized and was aggressive. She told us to begin letting other family members know and we should begin to say our goodbyes. What the oncologist told us was hard to swallow because in addition to her initial terminal diagnosis, Mom's cancer had returned twice in the previous five years and each time it returned, she overcame.

A few days after our heartbreaking conversation with Mom's oncologist, I took my dad to what I thought was a routine appointment with one of the specialists he sees. However, at the appointment, the specialist advised that my dad had cancer. I don't think it fully registered until they gave us the referral to an oncologist. Now Dad had radiation treatments to go to, in addition to appointments with his primary care physician, neurologist and urologist. Although, Mom's oncologist said there was not much more to be done, she decided to administer a small dose of chemotherapy to Mom, which meant that at the same time, she still had appointments to go to and not only with the oncologist, but the cardiologist, nephrologist and pulmonologist as well.

At this time, with both parents down again, all I could do was pray, pray and pray, which lead me to Psalm 121.

I will lift up my eyes to the hills—
From whence comes my help?
My help comes from the Lord,
Who made heaven and earth.
He will not allow your foot to be moved;
He who keeps you will not slumber.
Behold, He who keeps Israel
Shall neither slumber nor sleep.
The Lord is your keeper;
The Lord is your shade at your right hand.
The sun shall not strike you by day,
Nor the moon by night.
The Lord shall preserve you from all evil;
He shall preserve your soul.
The Lord shall preserve your going out and your coming in
From this time forth, and even forevermore.

Thank God for hearing my cry for help, because I didn't have to wait too long before He sent help our way.

After a few treatments of chemotherapy, Mom's oncologist and other providers determined that the treatments were not beneficial to Mom. The chemotherapy had a negative impact on other medical issues that Mom had contracted because of cancer. Mom appeared tired and everything became a struggle for her from bathing, dressing, eating to toileting. Mom was also often pleasantly confused. During some of Mom's confused states, she didn't know where she was, her name, her birthday, who the president was, where she was born and answers to other similar questions that used to come naturally to her and usually yielded a conversation, especially when she talked about where she was born and raised. That too was difficult for us to swallow because Mom had a career educating children and now she barely knew which state she lived in or the name of the President of the United States.

During the coherent states, which would abruptly come and go, and sometimes last for many hours or several minutes, Mom made it clear there were a few things she wanted to accomplish in the near future. One was to celebrate her and Dad's forty-ninth wedding anniversary with a homemade blackberry cobbler (I can't bake and neither could anyone close to us; as I previously explained, Mom was the baker, so we bought a blackberry cobbler from a local southern diner), celebrate her birthday with her nephew (who was the first in the family to share her birthday month) with cheese pizza from their favorite local pizza restaurant, make sure Dad was okay following his cancer diagnosis and treatments, and lastly vote, which was always something she was zealous about. If you allowed her to, she would share her thoughts with intensity on the importance of your vote and then quickly kick into educator mode and give you a history lesson on the Nineteenth Amendment and the Voting Rights Act of 1965.

At this point for Mom, we turned to comfort care, which meant she now needed twenty-four hour care. The good news at that time was Dad received his daily radiation treatments well. As I stated earlier, my brother and I worked, my son was in high school, therefore, neither one of us could be with Mom during the day. As a result of Mom's condition, she had a social worker who provided home health care options for us. A dear friend/sister I have known since I was nine years old had been recently laid off from her job at a pharmaceutical company, so she volunteered to sit in the interviews with the home health care providers with my parents, since she knew what to look for in a quality home health care provider. My dear friend/sister told me Mom made the interviews difficult. She didn't want "someone" in her kitchen, she didn't want "someone" washing their clothes, let alone washing *her*. As my dear friend/sister sat through the interviews, she had a revelation that truly blessed our family for the next three months. She decided since she was not working, she would become Mom's home health care provider during the day, which allowed my brother and me to continue our work schedules and resume caregiving duties in the evenings after work.

As I stated in Chapter Two, caregivers' roles and responsibilities will not remain the same; they change, as the patient's needs change. Comfort care is different from providing care for someone who is in treatment for a life-altering illness. Caring for the patient continues, however the caregiving goal is to make the patient comfortable as possible. Depending on the patient's disease, the end of their life may be years, months, weeks or days away. My thought for Mom at this time was to let her do exactly what she wanted and was able to do. So when Mom requested fried chicken at three a.m., followed by cheese pizza a few hours later for breakfast, we would do our best to get it for her, even though there was no guarantee she would eat it. Sometimes we could trick her into thinking she had the fried chicken she asked for by giving her french fries or a grilled cheese sandwich instead of cheese pizza. If Mom wanted to sit on "her" screened porch all day, even when it rained, she was able to do so. If Mom wanted to slide down the stairs on her behind because she didn't have the strength or energy to walk down the stairs, even with assistance, she was able to do so. At this point, Mom could not focus to read on her own, so we had to read to her, so if she wanted us to read something more than once to make sure she had an understanding of what was being read to her, we did so.

On one of Mom's hospital visits during this time period, she learned that one of her fellow church members and dear friend was also admitted to the same hospital on a separate floor. Mom demanded I take her to visit. She didn't care she was in the process of receiving medication from an IV and using a catheter. When the patient technician came to the room to take her vitals, Mom told her that I was evil because I would not take her to visit her dear friend. The patient technician explained to her that not only was she receiving medication by IV and had a catheter, but her immune system was low and if she visited another floor, she would expose herself to germs her body was not able to fight. Mom became more irritated with the patient technician than she was with me. Shortly after the patient technician left, the nurse assigned to Mom came in to issue another bag of medication through the IV. Mom pleaded her case with her nurse as well and the nurse too shut Mom down. Once the nurse left the room, Mom pressed the call button which sent the charge nurse to her room because she said as many times as Mom has been admitted and stayed on the oncology floor, she never complained and since she knew the nurse and patient technician assigned to Mom were currently caring for other patients on the floor, she came promptly to see what the problem was with Mom. I don't think the charge nurse had both feet in the room before Mom demanded they make a way for her to see her friend. Well, about thirty minutes later, the charge nurse came back and instructed me that I could actually take Mom upstairs to visit with her friend. She said she called the charge nurse on that floor to come in if we had not left within ten minutes. So with catheter and IV in tow, I was able to do what Mom wanted me to do and that was take her to visit with her friend.

Her friend was totally immobile; she had lost the use of her legs and she too had breast cancer as well as other medical issues. When we passed the nurses' station, they were aware of who we were and instructed the clock start ticking—fifteen minutes and counting because they figured it would take me about five minutes from that point to get Mom to the room. The ten minutes Mom spent with her friend felt like ten hours of bliss to each of them. They laughed, they reminisced, and they sang a portion of some of their favorite old church hymns such as: Pass Me Not, Because He Lives and His Blood Will Never Lose Its Power. Mom's fellow church member and friend did many things at the church well, but singing was definitely not one of them. To hear and see them so fragile and weak from their life-altering illnesses, but for those ten minutes be so happy and strong was truly a blessing, probably more for me than each of them. One thing that was clearly demonstrated during the ten minutes those two dear friends spent together was neither one of them had any doubt or fear about their current or future situation.

It is important for the caregiver not to feel as though they are giving up on the patient if the patient's prognosis yields to the last stage of the patient's life. As the caregiver, your role and responsibilities will become more intense, because not only are you still providing care for the patient, but you also have to deal with all that comes with anticipating the patient's death. If you have to choose hospice care for the patient, do not feel like you are giving up on the patient because you are not, you are making sure the patient is comfortable and pain-free until the end. At this stage in the patient's life, other individuals may become more involved in the patient's care such as home health aides, social workers, nurses, hospice care providers, nursing home workers, spiritual counselors, and pastoral staff. Hopefully, the patient previously prepared for the last stage of their life by doing some of the following:

1. Making their wishes known about their last stage of life in regards to treatment, whether they would like to be at home or in a medical facility at this stage. If the patient will spend their last stage of

life at home, the caregiver should ask themselves a couple of questions.

   a. Will the patient's home be able to accommodate a bedside commode, hospital bed and other medical equipment that may be necessary at this stage?

   b. Are you, the caregiver, mentally able to care for the patient at their home at this stage of their life? While you are caring for the patient at this stage, you will experience many emotions such as anger, anticipation, fear, grief, loneliness, relief and sadness.

2. Receive legal guidance and have documents such as a will, advanced directive (which provides details of the patient's desires for their health care and/or power of attorney).

3. Address and resolve conflict with family and close friends, so they will have peace and no regrets after the patient's death, because the conflicts cannot be resolved once the patient has passed away.

4. Expressed their desire about cremation or burial, what type of service or services they desire to have to celebrate their life.

If some or all the above are in place at this stage of the patient's life, then some of the caregiver's stress can be alleviated and they can better focus on caring and comforting the patient.

During the last stage of the patient's life, it is important for the caregiver to focus on the emotional care of the patient. The patient will probably be concerned, whether they express it verbally or not, about being a burden and losing control of their abilities as their health deteriorates. To comfort the patient, the caregiver should spend as much time as possible with the patient, whether there is conversation or not. Let the patient communicate their feelings even if they are hard to hear. Also, let the patient talk about their life, especially the good times because that will be comforting to the patient. To the best extent possible, make sure the patient maintains their dignity at this stage in their life.

One of my friends came to visit Mom to say "goodbye." However, at this stage in Mom's life, there was not much room for conversation with her because most of her hours were spent sleeping. Shortly after Mom acknowledged my friend's presence, she fell back asleep. My friend and I sat in Mom's bedroom talking about anything and everything but mainly reminiscing about our childhood and how we were raised. At one point in our conversation, my friend asked why God didn't heal Mom and she was at this unfortunate stage in her life. She also asked why God would allow such a caring, faithful, kind and rock to so many, suffer. Surprisingly, Mom answered faintly with fatigue in her voice and said, "My Jesus suffered; why shouldn't I?"

Then Mom fell back asleep. I didn't realize it then, but I realize now, Mom was healed when she transitioned, received her crown in Glory and the Lord said, "Well done, good and faithful servant" (Matthew 25:21).

Matthew 25:21: *"His lord said to him, 'Well done, good and faithful servant; you were faithful over a few things, I will make you ruler over many things. Enter into the joy of your lord.'"*

CHAPTER SEVEN

The Blessings

Galatians 6:9-10

"And let us not grow weary while doing good, for in due season we shall reap if we do not lose heart. Therefore, as we have opportunity, let us do good to all, especially to those who are of the household of faith."

God blessed me with two awesome parents. Being their caregiver provided me with the opportunity to not only get closer to them but to give back to them a portion of what they have given to me. Further, being their primary caregiver was a blessing because our family did not have to worry about the care my parents would receive if they were cared for by a formal paid caregiver our family did not know. In addition, being my parents' caregiver was a financial blessing, because our family did not have to pay for twenty-four hour care.

Although the activities of a caregiver are challenging, difficult and require a lot of energy they will bless you mentally, physically and spiritually.

I love my parents dearly, but being their caregiver forced me to serve them humbly in love. As a caregiver, you will be responsible for completing some unlovable tasks such as bathing and toileting, which were especially unpleasant for me after I let Mom eat whatever she wanted, but should not have done so. Especially when I was not up to a major bathing and toileting task.

Kindness, love, patience and understanding are essential characteristics when dealing with the challenges and difficulties of successfully performing caregiving duties.

As a caregiver, you must understand the patient's needs. For example, respect and understand the patient will not want to sit in soiled clothes, so you have to promptly be willing and able to care for their bathing and toileting needs. You must have serenity with the

The Blessings

patient. The patient may be angry and frustrated with you because you don't do things the same way or as quickly as a professional nurse, patient technician or home health aide, but you have to continue with the task you are doing; don't quit and take the time you need to complete the caregiving task even though the patient may be acting impatient and ungrateful. You have to always try to put yourself in the patient's shoes. As their caregiver, you are doing many things for the patient that they used to be able to do themselves. The patient is probably not happy about losing their independence; therefore, you must be tolerant and understanding.

Caregiving also requires analysis, complex thinking and multitasking because you have to handle the patient's financial matters, health insurance issues, medical needs and scheduling as well as your own responsibilities and commitments—all of which will provide you with plenty of opportunity to exercise your mind.

Caregiving requires physical movement because you will have to, among other things, lift, move and turn the patient and possibly climb up and down the stairs, all of which will provide good exercise for your body.

Throughout my life, I saw my parents live in a happy and healthy marriage to one another. The way my parents each lived their lives exhibited kindness, love and respect not only for one another, but also for everyone they encountered, which was always admirable to me. When disease struck, instead of being angry with God or at each other, both of my parents' faith increased and they appeared to trust God more than they previously had done, which was especially demonstrated in their marriage. Even with their limitations from their diseases, my parents remained devoted to each other, expressed tender care for one another, cherished each other more than they did in good days and good health and displayed unconditional love for one another in their actions and words. Living with a life-altering illness made my parents want to help others more than they did before their illnesses. They both appeared to understand other people's pain more than they did prior to their life-altering illnesses. My parents disregarded their own pain and wanted to help others the best they were able to do so with their limitations due to their health.

During Mom's battle with breast cancer, she always maintained faith, fight and victory. She was able to maintain victory because of her faith; she knew whether she survived cancer or died from it and went to heaven, she would win. Mom never complained. Not even when she had several procedures in a week, lost her hair and nails due to chemotherapy, gained weight from medication and couldn't wear her clothes or shoes, didn't have the strength to play her favorite hymns on her piano, cook for her family, travel with Dad, shop with her oldest grandson, play with her youngest grandson, bake with her nephew, hold her infant great-grandson, go to her favorite places: church, food, clothing and shoe shopping and the long trips to the bookstore. Instead of complaining, she continually thanked God for her bonus round. Mom was always concerned if the person caring for her had a good day. If they weren't, with her smile, words of wisdom and positive attitude she tried to do all she could to change their perspective. To Mom, that was more important than her care. She would say, "God has blessed me with good days, so I want you to have better days." Mom had a horrible disease, but still was never concerned about herself, only the well being of her family and friends.

My parents demonstrated while living with their life-altering illnesses that their tests were testimonies, which validated to me that Jesus is real. Their actions increased my faith and trust tremendously in the Lord and Savior, Jesus Christ. I also realized from my experience as my parents' caregiver that it is not the quality of my character that will bless me with the reward of heaven, but my faith. My caregiving experience has allowed me to truly relate to what Job said in Job 42:5: *"I have heard of You by the hearing of the ear, But now my eye sees You."*

Being a caregiver is challenging, difficult, stressful, takes courage as well as a lot of energy, but if you can do it, I believe the blessings of caregiving are priceless.

Acknowledgments

First, I would like to thank God for all He has done and continues to do in my life.

Secondly, I would like to thank God for helping me realize the blessings of caregiving.

Thank you Clifton Park Baptist Church for building my spiritual foundation and thank you, First Baptist Church of Glenarden under the leadership of Pastor John K. Jenkins, Sr. and his wife, First Lady Trina Jenkins for continuing to build on that foundation.

Thank you, Reverend Alethea Smith-Withers for allowing this caregiver to have a voice.

I thank God for blessing me with a loving, patient and supportive husband to share the rest of my life with, Robert Chappelle.

I would also like to acknowledge and thank those in my family, extended family and friends whose help has made this book a reality. Especially: Sam and Dada Akitobi, Mimi Beall, Inez Bregger, Mary Alice Bryant, Lynn Campbell, Faye, Hope and the late Georgia and Stanley (Jr.) Chappelle, Dwight, Kelli and Peggy Crutchfield, May Davis, Paris Davis-Reed, Lydia Dumas, Louise Gamble, the late Mary Pauline Garrett, Ed and Thelma Jackson, Carolyn, Tammy and the late Patsy Johnson, Karen Pearis Larenas, Glynn Lindsay, Cassandra Long, Chiner Long, Scott Long, Carletta Lundy, the late Larry "Stroll" Meades, Deborah McFadden-Lane, Artis and Juanita Palmer, Wendy Paulo, Pam Prue, Penny Prue, Tracy Debnam Staton, Jerome and Paula Stephens, Alice Ware, Astrid Ware, Susan Ware, Pamela Washington and Barbara Watson.